Ayurvedic skincare for men

*Discovering the ancient path
to radiant and healthy skin*

By Dr. Marcia Moss

Table of Content

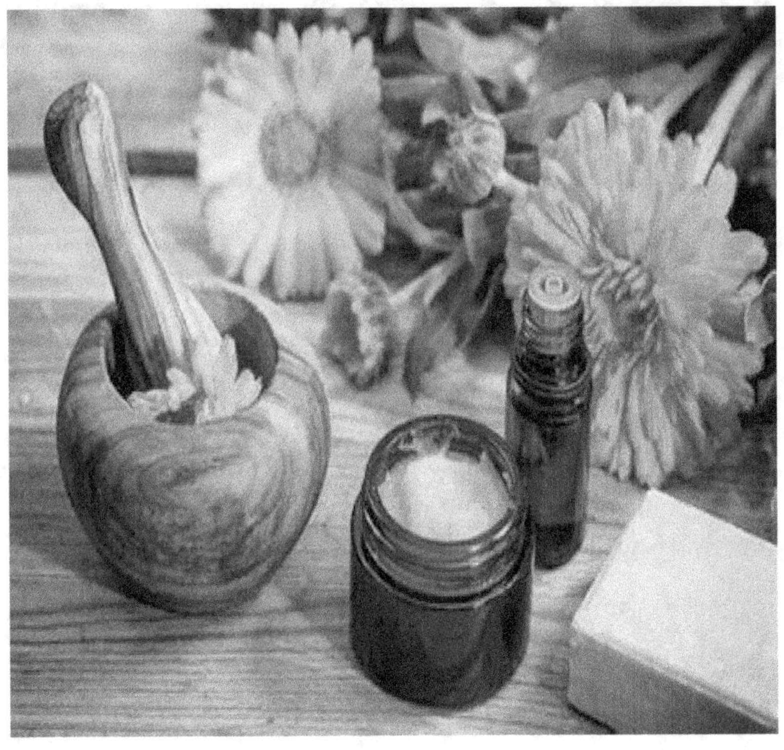

Chapter 1: Introduction to Ayurvedic Skincare

Welcome to the journey of discovering Ayurvedic skincare – a pathway to naturally radiant and healthy skin that has been cherished for centuries. In this chapter, we embark on a simple exploration of Ayurveda's timeless wisdom for achieving glowing skin that resonates with your unique self.

Ayurveda, an ancient Indian practice, teaches us to honor the delicate balance within our bodies and with nature. It believes that when we care for ourselves in harmony with our surroundings, our skin – our body's largest organ – reflects this harmony in its health and beauty.

Imagine Ayurveda as a guide, offering you gentle yet powerful insights into nurturing your skin. Rather than overwhelming you with intricate details, Ayurveda simplifies skincare into a joyful ritual. It's like weaving a tapestry of care that's easy to follow and embraces you like an old friend.

At the heart of Ayurvedic skincare are the doshas – Vata, Pitta, and Kapha. These are like your skin's unique personalities, each with its own qualities. Don't worry; this isn't a complicated process – it's a way to understand your skin better. It helps you know what suits it and what doesn't. It's like discovering the right rhythm for your skin's health.

Whether you're just starting or well along your skincare journey, Ayurveda embraces you. It's not about chasing trends; it's about embracing time-tested practices. It's about realizing that your skin, like nature, has its own seasons – sometimes it needs nourishment, sometimes detoxification. Ayurveda helps you listen and respond.

So, let's begin this journey with open hearts and curious minds. Together, we'll explore Ayurvedic skincare in a way that feels like chatting with a friend, sharing stories, and uncovering the secrets of vibrant, healthy skin. It's time to nurture your skin with love, and Ayurveda is here to show you the way – one simple step at a time.

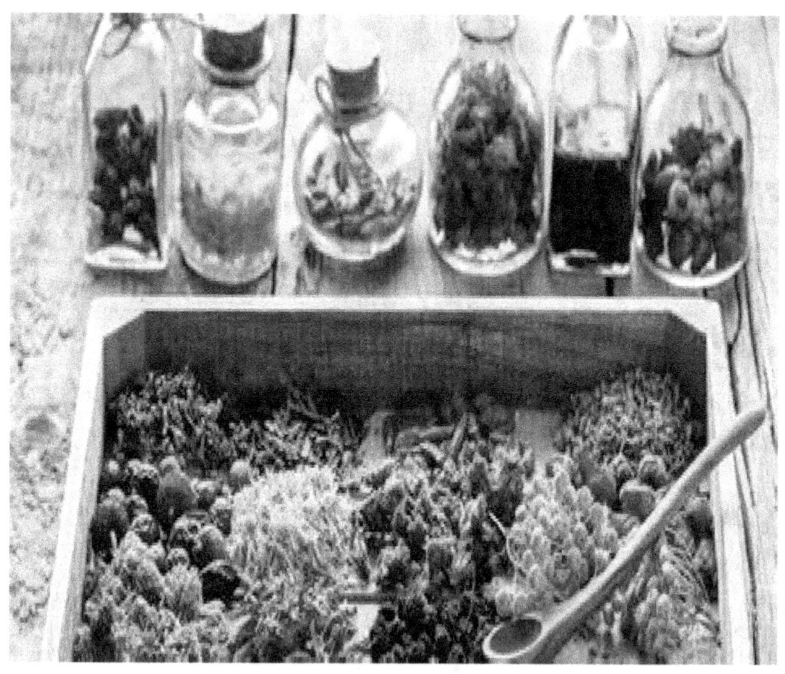

Chapter 2: Ayurvedic Wisdom and Your Unique Constitution

In the heart of Ayurveda lies an ancient wisdom that illuminates the path to radiant skin and overall well-being. Instead of diving into an intricate world of complex concepts, let's embark on a simple journey that reveals the essence of Ayurvedic principles and how they relate to your individual nature.

Understanding Ayurveda: A Friend to Your Skin

Imagine Ayurveda as your wise friend, offering insights into the tapestry of life, health, and skin. It views the body and mind as a harmonious whole, and by recognizing your unique constitution, you can uncover personalized ways to nurture your skin.

Doshas: The Building Blocks of You

Central to Ayurveda are the doshas—Vata, Pitta, and Kapha—like the primary colors that blend to create a masterpiece. Each person has a unique proportion of these doshas, shaping their physical and mental characteristics.

Vata: Think of Vata as the wind – creative, full of movement, and light. If you have Vata-dominant skin, it might be prone to dryness and quick shifts. You can support it with gentle care and nourishing routines.

Pitta: Pitta, akin to fire, is dynamic, passionate, and transformative. Pitta-influenced skin tends to be sensitive and reactive. Cooling and calming practices can help it glow with health.

Kapha: Like the earth, Kapha embodies stability, structure, and calmness. Kapha-related skin may lean towards oiliness and congestion. Invigorate it with lightness and invigorating activities.

Discovering Your Dosha

Determining your primary dosha is simpler than it seems. It's not a deep dive, but a gentle exploration. Reflect on your physical traits, preferences, and how you react to different situations. This helps unveil the shades of Vata, Pitta, and Kapha that make you, well, you.

Balancing Act for Your Skin

Picture doshas as musical notes, creating a melody of health. Sometimes, one note might play louder, causing imbalances. Ayurveda, like a soothing balm, guides you to bring harmony back.

By embracing the simplicity of Ayurvedic principles, you're embracing your skin's best friend. With this newfound understanding of doshas, you'll embark on a journey where the wisdom of Ayurveda merges seamlessly with your daily life, revealing a path to radiant and healthy skin that's uniquely yours.

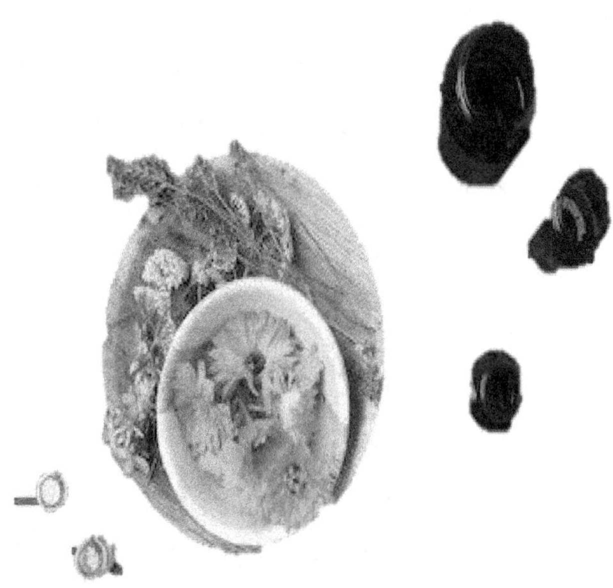

Chapter 3: Daily Skincare Rituals

In this chapter, we'll explore simple and effective daily skincare practices that seamlessly fit into your routine. Your skincare journey is like a journey through a garden, tending to your skin with care.

1. Gentle Cleansing: Start your day by cleansing your face with a mild, natural cleanser. This helps wash away the night and prepare your skin for the day ahead. A simple splash of water or a gentle cleanse with a soft cloth is all you need.

2. Hydration Harmony: After cleansing, hydrate your skin with a splash of cool water. It's like giving your skin a refreshing drink in the morning. You can also use a gentle, hydrating moisturizer that suits your skin type.

3. Mindful Massage: Take a moment to give your face a gentle massage. This isn't a complex tapestry of motions – simply use your fingertips to lightly tap and stroke your skin. It's like a friendly morning greeting for your skin.

4. Sunshield Love: Before stepping out, apply a natural sunscreen to shield your skin from the sun's embrace. Think of it as putting on your favorite cap to keep the sun from being too enthusiastic.

5. Evening Serenity: In the evening, treat your skin to another round of gentle cleansing. It's like a soothing bedtime story – preparing your skin for its well-deserved rest.

6. Calming Care: If your skin feels tired or stressed, apply a cooling gel or aloe vera. This simple gesture is like a hug for your skin, offering comfort after a busy day.

7. Restful Sleep: As you drift into slumber, your skin works its magic. Ensure you get enough restful sleep; it's your skin's time to rejuvenate and repair, just like a garden resting at night.

Remember, skincare isn't an intricate activity or a complicated journey. It's about these simple yet powerful rituals that speak the language of your skin. As you embrace these practices, you're embarking on a path towards radiant and healthy skin, the Ayurvedic way – like a kind friend guiding you on a gentle walk through a beautiful garden.

Your skin deserves this care, and these rituals are your way of showing it some daily love, like a warm hug that lasts all day long. So, let's continue this journey, step by step, with kindness and simplicity, nurturing your skin like you would a cherished garden.

Chapter 4: Nourishing Your Skin from Within

Our skin thrives when we give it the right nutrients from the inside out. Just like how a plant needs water and sunlight to flourish, our skin too needs nourishment to radiate its natural glow. This chapter is all about simple and effective ways to nurture your skin through what you eat and drink.

The Nutrient Connection:

Picture your skin as a canvas that reflects your inner health. What you put in your body really matters alot. Make the choice of a variety of fruits and vegetables.. They're like nature's vitamins for your skin, providing essential nutrients that help in maintaining its health. Think of carrots, bursting with beta-carotene, or juicy oranges loaded with vitamin C – they're like little beauty treats you can indulge in every day.

Hydration: Skin's Best Friend:

Keeping your skin hydrated is like giving it a refreshing drink. Water is the key to plump and supple skin. It's like nature's moisturizer that works from the inside. Aim for at least 8 glasses of water a day, and you'll notice how your skin thanks you with that healthy glow.

The Beauty of Balance:

In the world of Ayurveda, balance is everything. Just like life, your skin's needs change with the seasons. During colder months, warm, cooked foods can help your skin feel cozy and cared for. When it's warmer, embrace lighter foods like salads to keep your skin feeling fresh and vibrant.

Friendly Fats for Radiant Skin:

Not all fats are bad! Some are your skin's best friends. Omega-3 fatty acids, found in walnuts, flaxseeds, and fatty fish like salmon, are like little warriors protecting your skin's health. They keep your skin's barrier strong and help lock in that moisture.

Say No to Sugar Overload:

While an occasional sweet treat won't harm, too much sugar can be like a storm for your skin. It can lead to breakouts and dullness. Opt for natural sweeteners like honey or enjoy the sweetness of fruits without overloading on refined sugar.

Spices for Skin Health:

Spices aren't just for adding flavor – they're like secret ingredients for healthy skin. Turmeric, a golden spice, has anti-inflammatory properties that can calm irritated skin. Cinnamon can help regulate blood sugar, which indirectly benefits your skin's health.

Tea Time for Your Skin:

Sip on herbal teas like chamomile or green tea. They're like little potions with antioxidants that fight off free radicals, keeping your skin looking youthful and vibrant.

A Rainbow of Antioxidants:

Antioxidants are like shields for your skin, protecting it from damage. Blueberries, spinach, and even dark chocolate are packed with antioxidants that your skin will love.

The Joy of Mindful Eating:

It's not just about what you eat, but how you eat. Sit down, savor each bite, and give your body the time to digest. Mindful eating is a form of self-care that your skin appreciates.

Conclusion: The Skin-Nourishing Journey:

Remember, nourishing your skin from within is a journey, not a race. Small and consistency the key. Embrace colorful, whole foods, hydrate, and listen to what your body and skin need. By nurturing yourself inside, your skin will naturally reflect that care on the outside.

Chapter 5: Ayurvedic Herbs and Oils

In this chapter, we'll explore the wonderful world of Ayurvedic herbs and oils, nature's gifts for your skin's vitality. These natural treasures have been used for ages to enhance radiance and promote healthy skin. Let's dive in and uncover their gentle secrets.

Nurturing with Nature: Ayurvedic Herbs

Imagine your skin receiving a gentle embrace from Mother Earth herself. Ayurvedic herbs are like that embrace – tender and caring. These herbs are not some fancy potion, but the essence of plants that have stood the test of time. Their healing power comes from the wisdom of nature.

Aloe Vera – The Soothing Ally

Let's start with aloe vera, the friendly plant that's like a cooling breeze for your skin. Its gel is a go-to remedy for calming irritation and redness. Just a touch of it can make your skin feel as peaceful as a quiet morning.

Turmeric – The Golden Wonder

You've probably seen turmeric in your kitchen, but did you know it's a skin superstar too? This golden powder is like a sunbeam for your skin. It fights inflammation and helps your skin glow with happiness.

Neem – The Protector

Neem might not have the prettiest smell, but it's a guardian for your skin. This green gem fights off unwanted guests like bacteria and supports your skin's natural defenses. It's like having a loyal friend by your side.

Calming with Chamomile

Chamomile isn't just for tea. Its gentle nature is perfect for sensitive skin. It's like a cozy blanket that soothes and relaxes your skin, making it feel as calm as a tranquil sunset.

Reviving with Rosemary

Rosemary isn't just for cooking – it's a wakeup call for your skin too! This herb stimulates circulation, giving your skin a refreshing boost. It's like a brisk morning walk for your face.

Treasured Oils: Nature's Elixir

Now, let's talk about oils – nature's elixir for your skin. These oils are like a nourishing hug from the earth, keeping your skin soft and supple.

Coconut Oil – The Moisture Miracle

Coconut oil isn't just for pina coladas; it's a hydration hero for your skin. It's like a sip of water for a thirsty plant. This oil locks in moisture and makes your skin feel as smooth as silk.

Almond Oil – The Nutrient Booster

Almond oil is like a vitamin-packed smoothie for your skin. It's rich in nutrients that feed your skin's hunger for health. Imagine your skin getting a tasty treat that makes it glow.

Sesame Oil – The Rejuvenator

Sesame oil is like a fountain of youth for your skin. It's been cherished for centuries for its ability to rejuvenate and protect. Your skin will thank you as it gets a refreshing sip from this age-old well.

Gentle Massage: Your Skin's Daily Love

Now that we've met these incredible herbs and oils, let's talk about the art of massage. Massaging your skin isn't just about pampering; it's a way of saying "I care." Gently massaging with these herbs and oils is like a hug for your skin, improving blood flow and making your skin feel cherished.

In the next chapter, we'll bring it all together and guide you in crafting your personal Ayurvedic skincare routine. It's like creating a love-filled ritual that your skin will thank you for, every single day.

Remember, these herbs and oils are your allies on this journey to radiant and healthy skin. They're like the warm sunlight that kisses your skin, reminding you of nature's beauty and your skin's potential to shine.

Chapter 6: Addressing Skin Concerns using Ayurveda

Skin issues can be bothersome, affecting both your appearance and your confidence. Fortunately, Ayurveda offers gentle and natural solutions to tackle these concerns. Let's explore how Ayurvedic principles can help you regain healthy and radiant skin.

Understanding Your Skin

Before diving into remedies, it's important to understand your skin's behavior. Ayurveda categorizes skin into three types based on doshas: Vata, Pitta, and Kapha. Each type has unique characteristics that guide treatment approaches.

Balancing Vata Skin

Vata skin tends to be dry, sensitive, and prone to premature aging. To keep it balanced, favor nourishing oils like sesame or almond during massages. Use creamy, gentle cleansers that hydrate without stripping away natural oils.

Soothing Pitta Skin

Pitta skin is sensitive and can be prone to redness and inflammation. Cooling ingredients like aloe vera, cucumber, and chamomile can help soothe and reduce heat in the skin. Avoid harsh exfoliants and opt for gentle, calming masks.

Caring for Kapha Skin

Kapha skin is often oily and more prone to congestion. Light, non-comedogenic oils like jojoba or grapeseed can help. Regular exfoliation is essential to prevent buildup. Clay masks with antibacterial properties can be beneficial.

Acne and Blemishes: A combination of turmeric, neem, and honey can work wonders. Their antibacterial properties help clear the skin gently. Remember to cleanse, treat, and moisturize without over-drying.

Dryness and Flakiness: For dry skin, sesame oil massages (known as Abhyanga) can deeply moisturize. Hydrating foods like juicy fruits, nuts, and ghee can help restore moisture from within.

Eczema and Psoriasis: These conditions often result from imbalanced doshas. Applying coconut oil infused with calming herbs like licorice or calendula can provide relief. Focus on stress reduction and consuming anti-inflammatory foods.

Lifestyle Adjustments

Ayurveda emphasizes the mind-skin connection. Stress, inadequate sleep, and poor diet can contribute to skin problems. Incorporate stress-relief techniques like gentle yoga and meditation. Prioritize sleep and consume fresh, whole foods to nourish your skin.

Long-Term Care

Consistency is key. Follow a daily skincare routine tailored to your dosha. Use natural, gentle products that support your skin type. Regularly incorporate Ayurvedic herbs into your routine, like rose for soothing or neem for purification.

Seeking Professional Guidance

If your skin concerns persist, consulting an Ayurvedic practitioner can provide personalized guidance. They can assess your dosha imbalances and suggest targeted treatments, both internal and external.

Short Note

Ayurveda's approach to skincare is holistic, considering your unique constitution and the interconnectedness of your body, mind, and environment. By embracing these principles, you're not only addressing your skin issues but also nurturing your overall well-being in a natural and harmonious way.

Chapter 7. Lifestyle and Environmental Factors

Taking Good Care of Your Skin in Everyday Life

When it comes to achieving healthy and glowing skin through Ayurveda, it's not just about the creams and potions you put on your face. Your daily habits, routines, and the environment you're in play a significant role in the overall health of your skin. In this chapter, we'll explore some simple and practical steps you can take in your everyday life to support your radiant skin journey.

Balanced Routines for Radiant Skin

Creating a balanced daily routine is like giving your skin a steady rhythm to enjoy. Just like a well-choreographed activities, a consistent schedule helps your body and skin thrive. Wake up and go to bed at the same times each day to let your body's natural processes flow smoothly.

Nourishing Foods for a Nourished Complexion

Your diet acts as the canvas upon which your skin's health is painted. Embrace whole, natural foods that are rich in vitamins and minerals. Think of it as the colorful palette that can enhance your skin's natural beauty. Including fresh fruits, vegetables, and whole grains provides the nutrients your skin craves.

Shielding Your Skin from Environmental Stressors

Your skin faces a world filled with environmental challenges, much like a delicate tapestry in an open field. Protect it by wearing a gentle sunscreen when stepping out into the sun, and covering up in harsh weather conditions. This shields your skin from the elements and maintains its natural radiance.

Hydration: A Refreshing Drink for Your Skin

Picture your skin as a thirsty plant waiting for rain. Drinking water hydrates your skin from within, helping it stay supple and soft. Like quenching the thirst of a delicate flower, staying hydrated is a simple yet powerful way to keep your skin looking its best.

Stress Less for a Happy Complexion

Life's demands can sometimes create an intricate web of stress that affects your skin's glow. Think of stress reduction as a gentle journey you embark upon. Engaging in calming activities like meditation, deep breathing, or even a leisurely walk can help unravel the knots of stress, leaving your skin and mind refreshed.

Quality Sleep for Skin Rejuvenation

Sleep is like a comforting cocoon that wraps your skin in healing. Just like a caterpillar transforms into a butterfly within its cocoon, your skin undergoes repair and rejuvenation during sleep. Make sure to get your beauty rest, aiming for 7-9 hours of quality sleep each night.

Surrounding Yourself with Positivity

Your skin reflects the energy around you, much like a mirror that reflects light. Surrounding yourself with positivity and joy creates a beautiful aura that radiates through your skin. Spend time with loved ones, engage in activities that make you happy, and practice gratitude.

In essence, your lifestyle and the environment you choose to live in are the chapters that shape the story of your skin's health. By following these simple yet impactful practices, you're creating a beautiful narrative of radiant and healthy skin in your life. Remember, it's not about intricate steps, but about embracing the basics with a heart full of kindness and care.

Chapter 8. Holistic Wellness Practices

When it comes to having skin that glows and feels fantastic, it's not just about creams and lotions. We're about to explore a whole world of simple, everyday practices that can make a big difference in your skin's health and your overall well-being. These practices are like a secret toolkit that ancient Ayurvedic wisdom offers us.

Morning Refresh: Start your day with a smile and a refreshing routine. Before you dive into your day, try drinking a glass of lukewarm water. It's like giving your body a gentle wake-up call. You can even add a squeeze of lemon for a zing of Vitamin C!

Stretch and Move: Moving your body isn't about complicated activities or intricate routines. Just a few minutes of gentle stretching can get your blood flowing and your energy up. Maybe touch your toes, reach for the sky, or twist gently from side to side. It's like giving your body a warm hug to start the day.

Mindful Breathing: Take a moment to breathe deeply. Inhale through your nose, letting your belly expand like a balloon. let go of any stress by exhaling through your mouth,. It's like a mini-vacation for your mind.

Eat with Awareness: Food isn't just fuel; it's a way to nourish your body and skin. Try to eat your meals without rushing. Savor the flavors by chewing each bite slowly. It's like having a conversation with your food!

Nature Connection: Spending time outdoors, even if it's just for a few minutes, can do wonders. Take a walk, feel the sun on your skin, and listen to the sounds around you. It's like recharging your inner battery.

Digital Detox: We live in a digital world, but it's important to give your eyes and mind a break. Put your phone on silent, close your laptop, and just be. It's like giving yourself a little vacation from screens.

Gratitude Practice: Before you go to bed, think about three things you're grateful for. They could be big or small, like a delicious meal or a kind word from a friend. It's like tucking your heart in with a cozy blanket.

Gentle Movement: You don't need to embark on a hardcore workout. A simple evening stroll can be wonderful for your body and mind. It's like taking your mind for a walk too.

Peaceful Sleep: Your skin loves good sleep. Create a healthy and convenient bedtime routine that helps you unwind. Maybe read a few pages of a book or listen to soothing music. It's like giving yourself a sweet dream invitation.

Remember, these practices aren't about perfection. They're about adding little moments of care to your day.

Each one is like a stitch in the fabric of your overall well-being. And just like a cozy tapestry, these moments weave together to create a beautiful, healthier you.

In the next chapter, we'll dive into real stories of men who've embraced Ayurvedic skincare and wellness. Their journeys will inspire you to make these practices a part of your life too. So, let's keep things simple, friendly, and real – just like these holistic wellness practices.

Chapter 9. Transformations: Real Stories of Change

In this chapter, we'll share some remarkable real-life stories that demonstrate the genuine impact of Ayurvedic skincare on men's lives. These stories are like windows into the journeys of individuals who embraced the ancient wisdom of Ayurveda and experienced truly transformative results.

Story 1: Rekindling Confidence

Meet Samir, a young man who had struggled with persistent acne for years. His confidence was shaken, and he often felt self-conscious in social situations. Samir decided to explore Ayurvedic skincare as a last resort. By adopting a simple daily routine and incorporating skin-loving herbs like neem and turmeric, Samir witnessed a remarkable change. His acne gradually faded, leaving behind a newfound sense of confidence that radiated from within.

Story 2: Embracing Age Gracefully

John, a middle-aged man, had started noticing fine lines and dullness creeping onto his skin. Feeling apprehensive about the aging process, he turned to Ayurvedic principles. Through gentle self-massage with nourishing oils and a balanced diet tailored to his dosha, John's skin regained its vitality. While the wrinkles didn't vanish entirely, they told a story of a life well-lived, embraced with grace and care.

Story 3: Calming the Storm

Alex, an individual with sensitive skin prone to redness and irritation, had tried numerous products without much success. Frustration led him to explore Ayurvedic skincare, which emphasized the importance of understanding one's unique skin constitution. By using cooling and soothing herbs like aloe vera and chamomile, Alex's skin began to find balance. The redness gradually subsided, and his skin felt calm, like a tranquil sea.

Story 4: A Journey to Inner Radiance

Rajiv's story is one of overall transformation. Struggling with a hectic lifestyle and stress, his skin was a reflection of his inner turmoil. With the guidance of Ayurveda, Rajiv learned to prioritize self-care. Simple practices like meditation and mindful eating became his allies. As his mind found peace, his skin followed suit, radiating a healthy glow that mirrored his newfound inner serenity.

Story 5: Breaking Free from Harsh Chemicals

For years, Michael had been using commercial skincare products that promised quick results but left his skin dry and irritated. Seeking a natural alternative, he embraced

Ayurvedic principles of using gentle, nourishing ingredients. Gradually, his skin began to heal from the damage caused by harsh chemicals. Michael's story is a testament to the power of patience and the gentle touch of nature.

In each of these stories, the common thread is the simplicity and authenticity of Ayurvedic skincare. It's not about overnight miracles, but about embracing a holistic approach that respects the uniqueness of each individual's skin and life circumstances.

As you've seen through these stories, Ayurvedic skincare is a journey. It's a journey that doesn't demand perfection, but invites you to care for yourself with kindness and awareness. Just like these men, you too can embark on this journey, discovering the ancient path to radiant and healthy skin.

Remember, these stories are not about dancing with complicated routines or weaving intricate tapestries.

Instead, they're about embracing a straightforward and friendly way to care for your skin, making Ayurveda a part of your everyday life. Through these stories, we hope you find inspiration and courage to start your own transformative journey toward vibrant and authentic skin health.

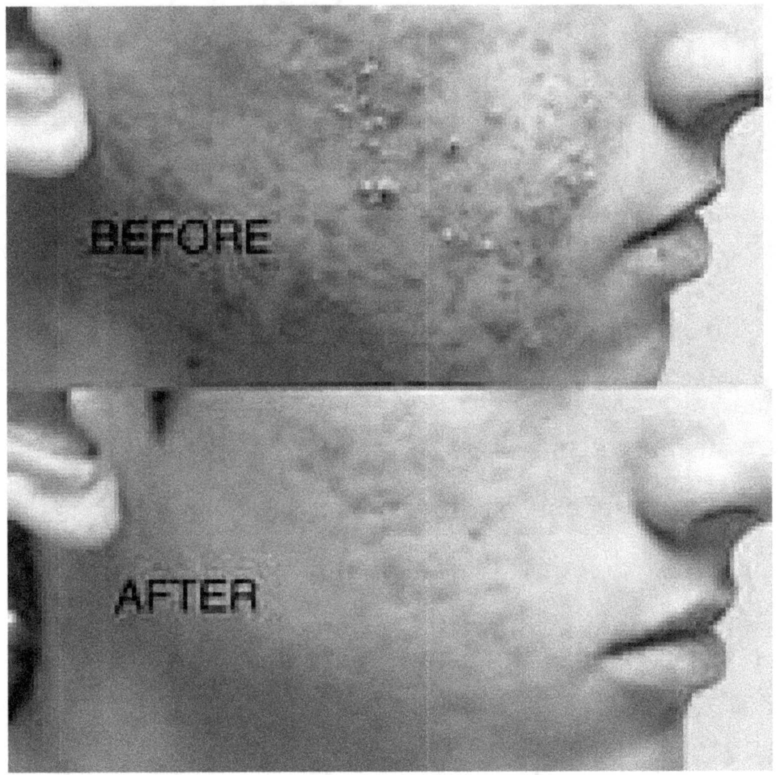

Chapter 10. Sustaining Your Ayurvedic Skincare Journey

As you've embraced the wisdom of Ayurvedic skincare and experienced its transformative effects, the journey doesn't stop here. Let's explore how to maintain your newfound radiant and healthy skin with simple, everyday practices. Remember, this is about making Ayurveda a harmonious part of your life, and it's as easy as a gentle breeze.

Consistency is Key

To sustain the glow that Ayurvedic skincare has brought into your life, consistency is your best friend. Just as the sun rises each day, keep up with your chosen routines. Be it morning rituals or evening self-care, let them become a soothing rhythm that your skin eagerly anticipates.

Listen to Your Skin

Your skin, like a close friend, communicates with you. Pay attention to its whispers. If it craves extra hydration, offer it a nourishing herbal infusion. Should it feel tired, treat it to a gentle massage with warm, fragrant oils. By tuning in and responding, you're nurturing a deep connection with your own body.

Nourish from Within

Remember, what you put inside shows on the outside. Feed your body with wholesome, nutrient-rich foods. Think colorful vegetables, juicy fruits, and whole grains. Sip on herbal teas that align with your dosha, infusing your cells with vitality and resilience.

Keep It Simple

In the world of Ayurveda, less can truly be more. Stick to the basics that have worked wonders for you. Simplicity is the beauty of Ayurvedic skincare.

Cleansing, moisturizing, and gentle exfoliation – these uncomplicated steps are your allies for sustained radiance.

Adapt to Seasons

Just as nature changes its colors, your skincare routine can evolve with the seasons. During colder months, provide extra moisture to your skin. When the sun shines, shield it from its rays and pamper it with cooling herbal masks. By attuning to nature's rhythms, you're ensuring your skin's vitality year-round.

Cherish Self-Care

Your skincare routine isn't a task to rush through; it's an act of self-love. Savor the moments as you massage your face with care, as you feel the textures of herbal concoctions on your skin. Every touch is an affirmation of your commitment to your well-being.

Connect with Others

Remember, you're not alone on this journey. Connect with fellow seekers of radiant skin. Share your experiences, learn from theirs, and create a supportive community. As you grow, your insights might inspire others to embark on their own Ayurvedic skincare adventure.

Your Personal Ayurvedic Sanctuary

Create a space where Ayurveda thrives. Arrange your oils, herbs, and skincare products in an organized, accessible way. This space isn't just practical; it's a reflection of your dedication to self-care.

Reflect and Rejoice

Pause to reflect on your progress. Take note of how your skin's texture has improved, how your confidence has grown. Celebrate every step, whether big or small. Your journey is a tapestry made of commitment and self-love.

Your Ayurvedic Journey Continues

As you conclude this book, remember that Ayurveda isn't a destination but an ongoing expedition. Every day presents a new opportunity to nurture your skin, honor your body, and celebrate the radiant glow that is uniquely yours. With Ayurvedic skincare as your guiding star, may your path be forever illuminated with health and vitality.

Thanks for Reading!

Dear Reader,

Thank you for embarking on this journey to discover the ancient path to radiant and healthy skin through the wisdom of Ayurveda. Your commitment to seeking natural and holistic solutions for skincare is truly commendable.

In this book, we've aimed to distill the essence of Ayurvedic principles into actionable steps that can transform your daily skincare routine. By understanding your dosha, nurturing your skin with herbs and oils, and embracing a holistic approach to wellness, you've taken a significant step towards nurturing not only your external appearance but also your overall well-being.

Remember, Ayurvedic skincare isn't just about looking good—it's about feeling good in your own skin. It's about honoring the connection between your body, mind, and spirit, and finding harmony within yourself and the world around you.

We hope the insights, activities, and practices shared within these pages become a source of inspiration as you embark on your Ayurvedic skincare journey. May your skin glow with health, radiance, and the timeless beauty that comes from embracing nature's wisdom.

With gratitude,
Dr. Marcia Moss